Low Fodmap Diet

A Comprehensive Guide To IBS-Acceptable Recipes With Fewer Restrictions For Digestive Wellness

(Delicious IBS Reliever Recipes To Beat Bloating And Soothe The Gut)

Ravinder Morrison

TABLE OF CONTENT

Introduction

My story leading up to this point is as follows: I have suffered from IBS and its various symptoms for a very long time, probably since the age of 2 6; I am now 6 8 years old, so it has been a while.

Over the years, I have visited countless doctors, taken countless expensive supplements, tried every diet, and undergone numerous medical tests in an attempt to determine what was wrong with me. I knew I had IBS, but I assumed it was something else because nothing I tried to fix it worked; however, nothing ever appeared. I wished something was actually wrong with me (obviously nothing serious) so at least I would know; I would have a solid reason for everything I was feeling, that it wasn't all in my head, and I could find the answers I was so desperately seeking.

However, this was not the case: none of the doctors, diets, tests, or supplements were effective. In addition to constant bloating, stomach cramps, and almost constant bad gas, I had both constipation AND diarrhea! Lovely!

As conventional medicine failed to provide me with the answers I sought, I became obsessed with finding a solution myself. I knew that gut health played an important role, so when I discovered that a plant-based diet can heal the gut microbiome, I was intrigued. I started watching vegan documentaries on

Netflix and reading vegan books by famous authors, and I became convinced that this was the solution to all of my problems.

As a meat eater, the idea of going vegan terrified me; giving up buffalo wings and cheese seemed absurd to me, but I had reached a point where I would literally try anything. I decided to really do a month-long vegan challenge - go completely plant-based and emerge transformed with a flat stomach, better digestion, and clearer skin, just as all the vegan influencers I followed said I would... However, that did not occur.

Chapter 1 : What Are Fodmaps?

A low FODMAP diet is also referred to as a FODMAP-free diet.

This is a temproraru eating rattern with a very low amount of FODMAP-containing foods.

The asronum represents:

- Fermentable substances are decomposed (fermented) by bacteria in the large intestine.

Oligo signifies "few" and "saccharide" refers to sugar. These molecules are composed of individual sugar molecules linked in a chain. This is a double molecule of sugar

- Monosassharides "mono" means single. This is a single sugar capsule.

- And Poluol are sugar alcohols (although they really do not cause toxicity!).

As you can see, your FODMAPs consist of four saccharide groups: oligosaccharides, disaccharides, monosaccharides, and polyols.

These FODMAP groups have distinct names and may contain more than one grain, known as FODMAP ubgrains:

- Olgoassharde have two ubgrour, referred to as frustan and galactans (or galasto-olgoassharde or GOS for hort).

- Dassharde are known as lastoe and constitute a single group

- Monoassharde are known as frustoe (or excessive fructose) and contain only one grain.

- Poluols contain two subgrours, sorbitol and mannitol

Let us examine the term FODMAPs, shall we?

The assharde and roluol are short-chain sarbohudrates that ferment in the lower part of the large intestine (bowel) if inadequately digested.

This fermentation process absorbs water and releases carbon dioxide, hydrogen, and/or methane gas, causing the substance to thicken and expand.

The result is severe diarrhea, abdominal distension, and other associated symptoms.

Chapter 2: What Is A Low Fodmap Diet?

The Primary Purpose Of This Diet Is To Alleviate Digestion-Related Symptoms, But It Is Also Proving Useful For Treating A Variety Of Other Conditions.

It Can Be Useful For Individuals With:

• Irritable Bowel Syndrome (Ibs) - See Below For Details.
• Additional Types Of Funtional Gastrointestinal Disorder (Fgid)
• Small 7ntetnal Basal Encroachment (Sibo)
• Certain Auto-Immune Sonditions/Diseases Like (Rotentiallu) Rheumatoid Arthritis, Multiple Sslerosis Or Eszema
• Fibromyalgia Or Other Health Issues Are Triggered By Particular Foods.

• Frequent Migraine Attacks That Recur After A Particular Meal
• Inflammatory Bowel Disease (Ibd) Includes Crohn's Disease, Ulcerative Colitis, And Multiple Sclerosis.

The Best Candidates For This Dating List Tend To Respond Affirmatively To These Questions.

Chapter 3: Low Fodmap Exercise Program

Can Exercise Help?

Irritable Bowel Syndrome is a greater issue than you may realize. It affects many people around the world. Some individuals with chronic problems and pain really do not associate it with certain foods. When they examine their bodies more closely, however, they realize that the bloating is caused by certain foods. These issues are caused by ineffective bowel movements. In some instances, their colons are simply too slow, while in others it is the opposite. It causes the colon to absorb either too much or too little fluid, resulting in diarrhea or constipation. I agree that eating the right foods is important, but regular moderate exercise is also crucial.

These are a few of the reasons why regular exercise will assist in alleviating these terrible symptoms:

Stress:

It is very well known that physical activity reduces stress. But how does this relate to IBS? IBS symptoms are strongly associated with stress. More than 98% of the time, your symptoms will worsen when you are exposed to stress. Due to stress, the nerves in the colon become extremely tense and cause abdominal pain. This is what causes the colon to become sluggish and causes the stomach pains in question. Aerobic and anaerobic exercise will both aid in the reduction of these symptoms. Walking, cycling, or working out for 6 0 minutes at the gym will release endorphins in the brain, thereby relieving tension in the bowls. The nerves in your colons will become more adaptable and efficient.

Some exercises, such as yoga, Pilates, and Tai Chi, involve breathing exercises. This is a regular occurrence for them. However, this should also be incorporated into your daily routine. These specific yoga deep breaths will increase your body's oxygen levels. Oxygen will eliminate any tension in your body, including the intestinal tension that is causing this issue.

Blood: Physical activity has numerous positive effects on the body. Not only does it help you lose weight and build lean muscle, but it also helps IBS patients by releasing tension and reducing stress. And this is essential for your condition. The sweating process will release so many toxins that will exacerbate your colon problems. By increasing blood flow, cardiovascular exercise will aid your bowel movements. With so many benefits associated with exercise, it is time to consider incorporating it into your daily routine. Harder to say than to do? I consent! However, I will attempt to offer some advice and inspiration on this matter...

Chapter 4: What Is The Function Of The Low-Fodmap Diet?

Many Americans view "diet" as a negative term because it evokes memories of starvation and arduous weight loss efforts. The low-FODMAP lifestyle differs from the majority of diets. It is a flexible eating plan designed to assist people with IBS, such as you or someone you care about, in making dietary changes that will improve their long-term health.

If you have IBS, you are already aware of its discomfort. Symptoms such as gas, cramps, bloating, and diarrhea can be both painful and humiliating. You may also have a lower quality of life because it is difficult to easy make plans when you really do not know if you will experience symptoms that require you to remain at home. With the low-

FODMAP diet, you can return to your life before you were diagnosed with IBS, free of stomach pain and embarrassment. It is an effective way to alter your lifestyle in order to feel better and simply reduce your symptoms.

The Scientific Foundation Behind FODMAPS

IBS is a functional bowel disorder, which means that there does not appear to be any anatomical, infectious, or metabolic issues; however, the symptoms persist and negatively impact the individual's health and quality of life. Since there is no clear cause for IBS, it is difficult for doctors to devise an effective treatment. Since no one knows for certain what causes IBS, most physicians treat the symptoms with medication, digestive treatments such as laxatives or bulking agents, and lifestyle advice.

In the 2000s, two researchers at Australia's Monash University wanted to determine if there was a connection between what IBS patients consumed and how they felt.

710 % of the research participants exhibited significant symptomatic improvement as a result of a particular eating strategy. You may experience a similar reduction or elimination of IBS-related discomfort by making the same deliberate dietary changes.

If you examine the list of foods that are high in FODMAPs, you may be curious about what these foods have in common. Both the high and low FODMAP food categories include both nutritious and unhealthy foods. The answer lies in the fact that they all contain carbohydrates.

Foods derived from plants are rich in fiber, simple and complex carbohydrates, and both. On the nutrition labels of packaged foods, simple carbohydrates are labeled as sugars, which can refer to either processed and refined sugars and syrups or sugars that occur naturally in milk, fruits, and vegetables. Complex carbohydrates are found in fruits, vegetables, grains, legumes, and legume products. They are sometimes referred to as "starch." Bacteria in the gut convert these carbohydrates into essential nutrients for our bodies.

Additionally, humans are unable to digest certain fiber-containing carbohydrates. Despite the fact that fiber does not provide the body with nutrients, it is essential for our health and digestion. It has been demonstrated that soluble fibers help maintain healthy levels of plaque and cholesterol. We have long recognized the ability of insoluble fiber to regulate bowel movements.

When they reach the digestive tract, these various forms of carbohydrates all begin to ferment. If something alters the number of active gut bacteria or the length of time a food spends in the gut, there may be a variety of consequences.

A person with a functional digestive disease may be unable to digest certain carbohydrates for a variety of reasons. For instance, their small intestine may lack sufficient bacteria or a particular enzyme. When carbohydrates are not digested in the small intestine, a condition known as malabsorption, the large intestinal bacteria suddenly have an abundance of the things they love to consume. Acids, alcohols, and carbon dioxide are byproducts of bacterial feasting, which is the same process that causes yeast to cause bread to rise or beer to be brewed. Having regard to this,

The gas is contained within the digestive system. Consequently, certain foods may cause you to feel and look bloated.

Even though this is already unpleasant, the situation worsens. As soon as fermentation begins, the pH of the gut is altered, which invites a plethora of additional symptoms, including gas and belching, inflammation, and acid reflux. The membranes lining the intestines and gut become permeable as a result of the rapid development of bacteria. Vital nutrients can escape the digestive system before being fully digested and absorbed.

These substances are also known as "osmotic" because of their ability to attract and retain water. The ability of sugar to attract and retain moisture is utilized by bakers and pastry chefs to keep baked goods moist and flavorful for an extended period. When a person sensitive to FODMAPs consumes sugar, they experience bloating and discomfort.

Even though the low-FODMAP diet has existed since 2002 , it has taken a while for research to demonstrate its benefits. A growing number of individuals, however, have found relief from their IBS symptoms by avoiding foods high in FODMAPs. Additionally, those with other conditions have benefited.

Chapter 5: Which Sibo Is Difficult To Treat

Typically, antibiotics are used to treat SIBO. However, studies indicate that recurrence develops in nearly half of all rats within a year of antibiotic treatment. A study comparing treatment with rifaximin (the most commonly used antibiotics for SIBO) and botanical antimicrobials revealed marginally better outcomes with the botanical protocol, but still effective treatment in less than half of all rats after a single treatment course.

These findings suggest that treating the overgrowth alone is insufficient for the majority of roles. Effective additional treatment must include addressing the underlying cause or predisposing factor.

Though numerous associations have been identified between SIBO and the diseases listed above, abnormalities in gut motility are recognized as one of the most common causes. One study published this month demonstrated that rats with SIBO have a significant decrease in small bowel transit time (the time it just take for something to move through the small intestine). This fndng suggsts that ratent with SIBO who really do not resover after a tandard soure of antbots or botanical antmsrobal rrotosol (which we prefer) may beneft from the addton of a rroknets agent that increases the muscular sontraston of the Ostreotide and low-dose naltrexone are two investigational drugs that may help treat some SIBO cases that really do not respond to antibiotics alone. Other treatments may include rrusaloride, low-dose erythromycin, and lubiprostone.

As research into SIBO continues, we are gaining a better understanding of the disease's complexity and how treatment must be individualized to maximize efficacy.

Chapter 6: What Is Irritable Bowel Syndrome?

To comprehend irritable bowel syndrome, we must take a brief trip through our digestive tract.

Human digestive system

Our digestive tract is composed of numerous organs. Its primary function is to digest food so that we can obtain the energy and nutrients we need to survive.

The digestive tract has its own nervous system, the enteric nervous system (ENS). It is responsible for the mixing and pushing of our food, as very well as determining what remains in our bodies and what is eliminated. This includes toxic and hazardous substances, with the immune system consulted.

The abdominal brain determines what we digest and keeps the digestive tubes open.

When the system becomes unstable

Because digestion is such a complex system, it reacts sensitively when one of its components ceases to function. In these cases, the body reacts negatively to food, resulting in gastrointestinal diseases. One of these diseases is irritable bowel syndrome (IBS).

Negative digestive tract reactions manifest as food intolerances and can be roughly categorized into two groups: food allergies and food intolerances.

Food allergy

The immune system overreacts to an innocuous foreign substance consumed via food. These hyperreactions are uncommon. The body behaves identically regardless of the amount of food consumed. The symptoms manifest all over the body, including swelling of the mucous membranes and tongue, nausea and vomiting, asthma, a runny nose, itching and eczema, and potentially fatal anaphylactic shock.

Food allergies

The immune system is not responsible. If you are intolerant, your body does not produce sufficient quantities of particular enzymes or proteins. As a result, some food components are incompletely digested. They are more prevalent, and the body's reactions vary greatly depending on the amount of substance consumed. The majority of the symptoms are limited to the digestive tract. Symptoms such as fatigue and headache are still possible.

Inflammatory bowel syndrome

However, irritable bowel syndrome can be triggered by food intolerance. IBS is one of the most prevalent digestive disorders.

Irritable bowel disease

Occasionally, IBS symptoms are mistaken for those of inflammatory bowel disease (IBD). The intestine repeatedly develops inflammation. This condition is characterized by diarrhea, bloody stools, stomach pain, abscesses, and fatigue. These diseases are most frequently represented by Crohn's disease and ulcerative colitis.

Since the symptoms of numerous gastrointestinal complaints are similar and the diseases are frequently misdiagnosed, it is crucial to consult a physician.

Avoid these foods if you're following a low-FODMAP diet: Meat: Beef, tuna in a can, chicken, deli slices made without high-fructose corn syrup (HFCS), fish, lamb, pork, shellfish, and turkey;

Lactose-free or low-lactose dairy products include cream cheese, half-and-half, hard cheeses (cheddar, Colby, parmesan, Swiss, etc.), mozzarella, sherbet, yogurt (Greek), and whipped cream.

Rice or almond milk alternatives, nuts (such as walnuts, macadamias, peanuts, pecans, and pine nuts), nut butters, tempeh, and soy milk derived from soy protein;

Gluten Grains: gluten-free loaves of bread, tortillas, cereals, portions of pasta, crackers, and chips made with spelled grains (corn, oats, potato, quinoa, rice, and tapioca), oatmeal and oat bran, popcorn, quinoa, rice, and rice bran; gluten-free loaves of bread, tortillas, cereals, portions of pasta, and crackers made with buckwheat grains (corn, oats,

Bananas, blueberries, cantaloupe, cranberries, grapes, grapefruit, honeydew, kiwi, kumquat, lemon, lime, mandarin, orange, passion fruit, pineapple, raspberries, rhubarb, strawberries, and tangerines; Alfalfa sprouts, bamboo shoots, bean sprouts, bell peppers, bok choy, carrots, cabbage, corn, cucumbers, eggplant, green beans, parsnip

Acceptable beverages include coffee, espresso made with lactose-free cow's milk, herbal tea (weak), dandelion tea, black tea (weak), green tea, peppermint tea, and white-leaf tea.

Chapter 8: Can Healing The Intestines Reverse Arthritic Symptoms?

The gut is central to the inflammatory response of the body. When there are mbalanse in the gut, it can boost the immune system and increase intestinal permeability, a condition known as leaky gut syndrome.

By restoring the balance of gut flora and enhancing the integrity of the gastrointestinal tract, arthritic symptoms usually improve. Leaky gut syndrome has been shown to be a key driver in autoimmune disease and to exacerbate inflammation.

How to better digestive health

Eating foods that nourish the gut lining, such as bone broths, stewed oxtail, and cabbage puree, is one way to alleviate digestive symptoms.

In addition, there may be foods that aggravate digestion and cause inflammation, such as tomatoes and citrus fruits, gluten, dairy, sugar, soy, red meat, and alcohol. Following an elimination protocol can help identify food sensitivities, or you can use food sensitivity testing to determine which foods may be problematic for you.

Not only does it matter what you eat, but also how you eat. Proper digestion requires that you practice mindful eating, chew food thoroughly, and eat in a retracted position. Take time before a meal to breathe deeply and feel gratitude, and then consume the food with all of your senses.

Immune and joint health are dependent on the health of the gastrointestinal system. Take a functional medicine approach to your healing and work upstream to improve your symptoms, as opposed to focusing solely on your symptoms. Not only will you feel better, but you may also find that by working on your gut, your symptoms improve over time.

The 7-Day Low FODMAP IBS Diet Plan Absolutely Required Reading Before Beginning:
• Consult your doctor or dietitian prior to making any changes to your diet or exercise regimen. While I am a qualified dietitian, I am unfamiliar with your personal medical history, your current medications, and any other relevant factors.

• This diet is extremely restrictive and only temporary: A low FODMAP diet is extremely restrictive and is not appropriate for those who are not following it for medical reasons. It is also a temporary eating pattern comprised of the Elimination Phase (2 st) and the Reintroduction Phase (2nd); you can learn more about it here. This strategy focuses on the Elimination Phase.

• Unsuitable for certain medical conditions, including people with diet-related medical conditions (such as type 2 or type 2 diabetics taking medication) and those at risk for developing eating disorders or emotional instability. Moreover, any elimination diet for a child must be carried out under the direct supervision of a dietitian.

• Download this list of low-FODMAP foods. Important portion size because the majority of low-FODMAP foods still contain small amounts For example, a serving of pineapple has a low FODMAP count, but if you consume half a pineapple at once, your FODMAP intake will increase. Download this list as a guide to low-FODMAP foods.

• Choose water as your beverage of choice; alcohol is not included in the meal plan, so keep a bottle of water with you at all times. Black coffee, black tea, peppermint tea, and green tea contain negligible amounts of FODMAPs and are safe to consume (no milk).

• Prepare all meals at home whenever possible. Typically, avoiding unintentional consumption of high-FODMAP foods requires advance meal planning, which is why I recommend downloading the shopping list for each week's worth of recipes at the bottom of this post.

• Keep a food journal: Record every meal you consume along with any negative symptoms you experience immediately following each meal or later in the day. This is known as a food diary and is essential for identifying triggers and preparing for the reintroduction phase. Here is a simple example from the Healthy Food Guide New Zealand that you can copy, or you can simply write your own at home.

When preparing your grocery list, keep in mind that the majority of your recipes yield between two and four servings. You will have surplus food. Feed the family or save the leftovers for a meal on another occasion.

EATING OUT

How really do you navigate dining out while adhering to a low-FODMAP diet? The following recommendations apply:

810 . ONLINE MENU CHECK

Always check the menu online first. Certain restaurants are notoriously difficult to find low FODMAP alternatives at.

You can determine if the restaurant has any options for you by viewing the online menu.

86. FOR MORE INFORMATION ON THE OPTIONS, CONTACT THE RESTAURANTS.

Once you've decided on a restaurant, give them a call and let them know what your main food allergies are. Inquire as to whether this can be accommodated.

When calling a restaurant, you can frequently find out how seriously they take your sensitivity, which can help you decide whether or not to dine there.

87. SELECT DISHES THAT APPEAR SAFE AND ADAPT THEM

If you arrive at a restaurant without a reservation, it is prudent to select the dish that appears to be the most secure. Steak served with fries and a salad, for example.

Then, inform them of your intolerances, inquire about the dish's ingredients, and request that any necessary substitutions be made.

On this basis, you and the restaurant staff can create your own low-FODMAP cuisine.

88. WATCH HOW MUCH YOU EAT.

IBS patients may experience symptoms after an excessive meal. Therefore, it is prudent to monitor your portions when dining out.

Try to eat slowly, thoroughly chew each bite, and stop when you are full. Despite the fact that this is not always possible, it is still wise to be aware of it.

The diet is low in FODMAPs, not FODMAP-free.
Remember that this diet emphasizes consuming low-FODMAP foods rather than avoiding them entirely. This gives you a little bit more freedom in a restaurant.
However, most people only need a small amount of garlic or onion to experience symptoms, so be mindful of your trigger foods.

LACTASE SUPPLEMENTS CAN BE USED TO INCREASE LACTASE TOLERANCE

When consuming a meal containing lactose, lactase pills are available for purchase.

This supplement will help your body break down lactose, allowing you to consume lactose-containing foods without difficulty. This information may save your life in a restaurant!

Chapter 9 : The Low-Fodmap Diet

In essence, a diet low in FODMAPs is an elimination diet. In addition to the allergy elimination diet, there are the keto, paleo, and autoimmune paleo diets (AIP). The objective of all elimination diets is to simply reduce or eliminate specific foods or food groups that may be the cause of specific reactions or symptoms. Later, you may reintroduce these foods or increase your consumption of them to determine which ones negatively affect you or, in the case of many elimination diets, increase autoimmune markers and flare-ups. Frequently, a low FODMAP diet is prescribed to treat irritable bowel syndrome (IBS) or small intestinal bacterial overgrowth (SIBO).

What to Select (LOW-FODMAP)

Naturally, many foods are low in FODMAPs. Here is a list of low FODMAP-friendly foods (10 Trusted Sources, 6Trusted Sources):

Beef, chicken, eggs, fish, lamb, pork, prawns, tempeh, and tofu are sources of protein.

White and brown rice, lentils, corn, oats, quinoa, cassava, and potatoes are examples of whole grains and starches.

Blueberries, raspberries, pineapple, honeydew melon, cantaloupe, kiwi, limes, guava, starfruit, and strawberries are examples of fruit.

Bean sprouts, bell peppers, radishes, bok choy, carrots, celery, eggplant, kale, tomatoes, spinach, cucumber, pumpkin, and zucchini are examples of vegetables.

Almonds, macadamia nuts, peanuts, pecans, pine nuts, and walnuts (no more than 2 0 per sitting).

Seeds: pumpkin, sesame, and sunflower seeds, as very well as linseeds

Lactose-free milk, Greek yogurt, Parmesan, Colby, cheddar, and mozzarella cheeses are dairy products.

Coconut and olive oils are examples of

The drinks are peppermint tea and water.

Cumin, saffron, cinnamon, paprika, coriander, cardamom, soy sauce, fish sauce, certain chile-based products, ginger, mustard, pepper, salt, white rice vinegar, and wasabi powder are some of the condiments used.

Although coffee, black tea, and green tea are all low FODMAP foods, caffeinated beverages are typically discouraged on a low FODMAP diet because caffeine is a common IBS trigger.

Chapter 10: Ibs: Its Origins And Diagnosis

Possible causes include an overly sensitive colon and an immune system. Post-infectious IBS is caused by a previous bacterial infection of the gastrointestinal tract. The shifting potential causes easy make it difficult to prevent IBS.

According to studies, the colon is easily affected, going beyond mild excitement. Instead of slow, rhythmic muscle development, the entrail muscles are fit. This may result in diarrhea or clogging.

One more hypothesis suggests that it may contain body-made synthetics, such as serotonin and gastrin, which regulate nerve signals between the brain and gastrointestinal tract.

Diet is the reason for deteriorating stomach health.

Dairy is the most well-known food prejudice, affecting a quarter of individuals who have analyzed or are aware of their food prejudice. 2 0-20% of individuals have a sensitivity to wheat, gluten, or lactose.

Possible causes include:

Broken stomach-brain communication, which can be influenced by stress and anxiety: The brain and the stomach are (naturally) different sides of the same organ; they develop from the same precursor cells, so if you dislike the brain, you're likely to have stomach problems, and vice versa. This is clinically evident. People with mental illnesses, such as depression, anxiety, PTSD, and neurological conditions, such as Alzheimer's disease and Parkinson's disease, are likely to have gastrointestinal issues. Additionally, individuals with chronic gastrointestinal illness, such as inflammatory bowel disease (Crohn's disease and ulcerative colitis), irritable bowel syndrome, or celiac disease, are likely to have neurologic and mental issues, such as anxiety, depression, and PTSD."

Earlier stomach diseases or food contamination: "This is known as post-irresistible IBS, and it can occur out of the blue following a stomach contamination. It may take a very long time for a persistent condition to disappear.

Hereditary traits: If IBS runs in your family, you are likely to develop it sooner or later, although not in the sense of an immediate inheritance.

Awkward stomach microorganisms or an overabundance of microorganisms in the small intestine (SIBO); changes in stomach "motility," also known as how quickly or slowly food and waste travel through the intestinal system; and finally, innate extreme sensitivity, as in delicate nerves in the GI tract.

Diagnosis

There is no test for IBS, but you may require a few tests to rule out other potential causes of your symptoms.

Your medical service provider will likely begin with a comprehensive medical history, physical exam, and tests to rule out other conditions, such as celiac disease and inflammatory bowel disease.

Your primary care physician (PCP) may ask you the following:

What types of gastrointestinal adverse effects are you experiencing?

How frequently really do you experience side effects? They return and forth, or really do they occur consistently?

Are certain foods responsible for specific side effects?

Really do you observe side effects during or after periods of stress?

Really do you have a history of IBS or other gastrointestinal disorders in your family?

The FODMAP elimination diet is the most effective method for detecting and diagnosing irritable bowel syndrome (IBS).

FODMAP is an acronym for fermentable oligosaccharides, disaccharides, monosaccharides, and polyols, which are short-chain carbohydrates (sugars) that are poorly absorbed by the small intestine. Some individuals experience stomach-related issues after consuming them.

The low-FODMAP diet temporarily restricts these starches to alleviate uncomfortable side effects and rest your stomach-related framework.

Chapter 11: Implementation Guidelines

In daily life, it is not always simple to strictly adhere to a list of acceptable food sources. Whether it is a business dinner, a gathering with friends, or a family outing to a café, dining out is a common occurrence. Initially, only one out of every odd restaurant has acceptable dishes that FODMAP-reduced acquaintances may enjoy. It means eating regimen for you. Even acquaintances and you must design a great deal in order to know which foods are acceptable, particularly at the beginning of your diet change. This piece can be depleting in the beginning. But really do not let this depress you. You will quickly become accustomed to your new diet and will soon be able to deal with it routinely and without stress.

Obviously, you can inform your family in advance which food sources you can tolerate and which you cannot. Assuming that your companions are somewhat perplexed, you can send them a couple of recipe suggestions to ensure that nothing disrupts the general flow of a pleasant dinner together. Perhaps you should first invite your loved ones to your home and prepare a divine meal. Thus, you can persuade everyone that FODMAP-friendly dinners are also incredibly delicious, given that generally uninvolved individuals have a few reservations about trying new foods. You will see, however, that the others will be quickly persuaded that this type of diet also offers delicious meals.

The situation may become more difficult in the restaurant. Assuming you sit in a café and peruse the menu for the third time in search of dishes that are suitable for you, this can quickly become awkward and stressful. You should be able to enjoy a meal at the restaurant without having to search for a suitable dish. Currently, the majority of menus are also accessible online. Therefore, investigate the menu at home to avoid unnecessary pressure in the café. You may have successfully located something and can now casually anticipate your visit to the restaurant. If you haven't found what you're looking for, call the restaurant and briefly explain your issue. For what the culinary expert can provide or prepare based on your preferred food types. You can also send a brief email if you intend to visit a restaurant a few days later. In the best case scenario, you should share all food sources that you can tolerate very well and that the chef can use to create an exceptional dish for you. Generally, restaurants will come to you and serve you a prearranged meal or two. Later, simply let us know which day you will be visiting so the easy cook can be prepared.

There are certainly cafés that are more understanding of your situation than others. It is advisable to keep track of all cafés and your involvement in relation to them. Assuming you have a business lunch or dinner with friends, you have a list of restaurants from which you can choose. Your coworker has no idea why you're recommending one of these restaurants so that a terrible situation does not occur. Your companions will be pleased that you can finally return to a restaurant for a casual dinner with minimal difficulty.

In the private sector, it is advantageous if, prior to going out to shop, you carefully consider which meals you will need to prepare at home within the next few days. After deciding on all of the appropriate dishes, you should create a shopping list. This prevents you from remaining in the store without knowing precisely which food sources you are allowed to consume. In addition, you go shopping with a list and avoid temptations that could derail your diet. With this method, you also prevent unnecessary extras from becoming trash. Assuming you plan ahead, you can prepare meals for the following days so that you can consume all the food.

Chapter 12: Lists Of High And Low Fodmap Foods

Which food varieties are high and which are low in FODMAPs? These two lists can help you determine which food sources to eliminate during the initial phase of your diet and which you can keep when planning the remainder of your meals and snacks. If you really do not know about a food, investigate it. You may also notice that a "sufficient" food is bothering you; try eating less of it or eliminating it entirely.

Depending on where you look, you may find seemingly contradictory data (for example, coconut appears on both a list of high FODMAP and low FODMap food varieties), but this generally indicates that the asset is referring to a specific section. A quarter-cup of shredded coconut is considered low in FODMAPs, but any more and you'll consume an excessive amount of polyols. If all else fails, investigate a specific food and determine if you're eating excessively. Additionally, remember that just because a food is acceptable in one structure does not mean it is acceptable in all structures. Using coconut as an example once more, a quarter cup of shredded coconut is low in FODMAPs, whereas a single serving of coconut water is high.

Chapter 13: What Foods Are Permissible On A Low Fodmap Diet?

The average FODMAP intake from a regular or high FODMAP diet ranges from 0.10 to 2 ounce (2 10 to 6 0 grams) per day.

Converelu, a low FODMAP det am to lmt your ntake to 0.02 ounces (0.10 grams) per meal — an extremelu low amount that translates to 0.08–0.2 ounces (2.10 –6 grams) per meal if you eat small, frequent meal. Fortunately, numerous foods are naturally low in FODMAPs. Here is a list of foods you may consume while adhering to a low FODMAP diet:

* Proten: beef, shaved venison, eggs, fish, foie gras, lamb, rork, rrawn, tempeh, and tofu

* Complete grains and starches: white and brown rice, linseed, spelt, oats, quinoa, cassava, and potatoes

* Frut: blueberries, raspberries, rnearrle, honeydew melon, santaloure, kiwi, lme, guava, starfruit, and grapes * Bean rrout, bell rerrer, radhe, bok shou, sarrot, seleru, eggrlant, kale, tomatoe, rnash, susumber, and pumpkin Almond (no more than 2 0 at a time), masadama nut, reanut, resan, pine nuts, and walnuts.

* Seeds: pumpkin, sesame, and sunflower, as very well as flaxseed Lactose-free milk, Greek yogurt, Parmesan, Colby, cheddar, and mozzarella cheese. Coconut oil and olive oil * The replacement beverages are tea and water. Sumn, affron, cinnamon, rarrka, sorander, sardamom, ou ause, fish sauce, some chile-based seasoning. rrodust, gnger, mutard, rerrer, alt, white rice wine vinegar, and waab rowder

While coffee, black tea, and green tea are all low FODMAP foods, caffeinated beverages are typically discouraged on a low FODMAP diet because caffeine is often an IBS trigger.

In addition, it is essential to check the ingredient list on packaged foods for FODMAPs. FODMAPs may be added to foods for a variety of reasons, including as preservatives, fat substitutes, or low-calorie sugar substitutes.

Soaked Oats Porridge

Ingredients:
- 1/2   teaspoon salt
- 2 tablespoon olive oil or butter
- fresh lemon juice (optional)

- 2 cup old-fashioned oats
- 2 cup milk

Instructions:

1. Rinse the oats in a fine mesh strainer.
2. Add them to a medium saucepan with the milk and salt.
3. Easily bring the mixture to a boil over medium heat, stirring frequently.
4. Simply reduce the heat to low and simmer, stirring occasionally, for about 25 to 30   minutes, until the oats are soft and creamy.
5. Remove the pan from the heat and stir in the olive oil or butter.

6. Serve warm, topped with a sprinkle of lemon juice if desired.

a Few Suggestions Before Beginning The Low-Fodmap Diet

Begin by collecting and experimenting with recipes. This is essential, as it will prevent you from preparing numerous subpar meals. Begin by collecting and testing recipes so that you have at least five that you can easy cook whenever you're hungry.

Keep a food journal

Obtain a diary or journal to record your diet. It may sound tedious, but it's important so that you don't become too arrogant after not experiencing your usual stomach cramps and then proceeding to eat dinner. Therefore, keep records because they will be extremely useful. Additionally, this could serve as motivation by reminding you of where you started and how far you've come.

Maintain an open mind.

You will be pleasantly surprised by the results of experimenting with new recipes. Abandon your preconceived notions, be subjective rather than objective, experiment, be your own scientist, and maintain an open mind.

Identify a term for low FODMAP

This is not a common form of diet, so get a brief explanation whenever you're out, particularly if you're the social type. It is easier and less embarrassing if you have a concise explanation for situations, so that your digestive system is not the subject of a lengthy discussion.

Seek advice from a dietitian

Seek professional assistance to determine whether you have an underlying medical condition.

...........Don't Panic

Some individuals are devastated to discover that they cannot consume any of the foods they adore. Please really do not be alarmed that the beginning is quite terrifying.

.easy cook

Chapter 14: Some Suggestions For Managing Ibs

This section will discuss IBS management strategies in general.

Meditation

Meditation is one of the strategies for managing IBS in general. Currently, many individuals really do not fully comprehend how mediation works. They believe that meditation entails nothing more than sitting in silence and thinking of nothing. Therefore, to them, it sounds extremely dull.

However, the reality is that meditation is quite different from sitting still and thinking of nothing.

Meditation involves being present in the present moment. Take note of the thoughts in your head, the rumbling sounds in your stomach, and your heartbeats.

A few days of regular meditation, even if only for 510 minutes per day, will significantly reduce your overall anxiety levels and easy make you feel more relaxed.

If you find the idea of formal meditation tedious, you can incorporate meditation into your life in alternative ways.

A great way to achieve this is to prepare and enjoy a meditative cup of tea in the morning, followed by a quiet excursion to enjoy it. Before drinking the tea, inhale its aroma and observe its quality and hue. Additionally, thank you for the cup of tea in front of you. And when you really do consume the tea, savor each sip.

Consider the sensation of a warm liquid moving down your throat and settling in your stomach. Take the time to appreciate and be present with the tea.

Consume foods containing Probiotics

It is also beneficial to consume a diet rich in probiotics if you suffer from IBS. The most effective probiotic foods are fermented foods. Our digestive system is typically stressed, and when it is, it requires a high probiotic concentration.

If you continue to take probiotics regularly, you will experience more regular bowel movements than you are accustomed to. As a vegan, it is essential to read the label of every probiotic supplement you purchase because not all were designed with vegans in mind.

Numerous probiotic supplements contain dairy, which is incompatible with veganism.

For the majority of IBS sufferers, the diary is off-limits. Due to my severe lactose intolerance, I was forced to give up the ice cream that I enjoyed so much.

If you have IBS, I recommend keeping a food journal for at least one week.

Record everything you consume, including every meal, snack, and nibble. In addition, record the exact timing of these meals and the symptoms you typically experience after consuming them.

You will then be able to identify the foods that are causing your IBS symptoms and eliminate them from your diet gradually. If chocolate is your trigger food, you must be willing to eliminate it from your diet. This elimination is not, however, permanent. You will not eliminate it permanently. You will only eliminate it from your diet for a few weeks before reintroducing it gradually to observe the results. And the same holds true for every food you eliminated from your diet.

You are eliminating the food from your diet and reintroducing it after a few weeks to ensure that it is the food and not stress or your monthly cycle that is causing your IBS symptoms.

Add more fiber to your diet gradually.
A deficiency in dietary fiber may be one of the causes of digestive problems such as irritable bowel syndrome. Fiber aids in maintaining a healthy digestive tract. Unfortunately, the majority of Americans today really do not consume enough fiber daily.

Consider that the amount of fiber you add to your diet will depend on the severity of your IBS symptoms at the time.

There are typically two types of fiber: soluble and insoluble.

Soluble Fiber

Soluble Fiber works by slowing down the digestive process. Thus, it is beneficial for someone who has diarrhea. The most popular sources of this type of fiber are oats, butternuts, squash, and chia seeds.

Insoluble Fibrous Substances

The following fiber type is insoluble fiber. Vegetables, legumes, whole grains, and legumes all contain this type of Fibre. They stimulate the digestive tract, making them an ideal addition to anyone's diet.

If you suffer from chronic constipation, you must include this type of fiber in your diet.

And it is beneficial to begin slowly. Start with 1525 tog of fibers and gradually increase to 48,510 tog. If you really do not really do it this way, you will struggle to adapt to it. You will also experience unbearable gas, bloating, and stomach cramps, which you should avoid.

really do really do really do really do

Chapter 15: Ways To Increase Plant Consumption On A Low Fodmap Diet

BAKE: low FODMAP breakfast muffins and store them in the freezer for a midnight breakfast with no need to wake up early. Find buckwheat breakfast pancakes on the website modernguthealth.com.

Combine one serving of rnash (or kale) with one to two servings of almond, rye, or hemp beverage. Utilize in hot cereal, granola, pancakes, crepes, muffins, smoothies, and curry.

CEREAL: Add 1/2 cup of shredded carrots or zucchini to hot cereal (oatmeal, buckwheat, teff, millet, quinoa, rice) or overnight oats with cinnamon and maple syrup.

CHIPS: easy make srisru baked vegetable shirs: carrots, kale, rarsnirs, plantains, rotatoes.

GRANOLA: Prepare a double batch of low FODMAP granola in less than thirty-six and zero minutes. Examine my recipe in the morning.

GRATE: Utilize the attachment on your food processor that shreds vegetables. Try sardines, cucumbers, or zucchini and store them in the refrigerator for use in a salad throughout the week.

Low FODMAP nuts and seeds can be ground into a flour that can be added to cereal, yogurt, smoothies, or to replace bread crumbs.

PESTO: Use leftover greens (spinach, arugula, kale, rarleu, cilantro, mint), low FODMAP nut (walnut or rne), and garls-infused oil in place of garlic. You can substitute nutritional yeast for parmesan. Freeze in ice cube traus.

SAUTÉ: sauté low FODMAP greens such as chard and kale for 12 to 2 minutes and bok choy and collard greens for 8 to

12 minutes. Utilize soy sauce or tamari to season.

It is enjoyable to consume zusshn noodles either hot or cold. Try it with red and sun-dried tomatoes.

Chapter 16: Almond-Stuffed French Toast

Moderate FODMAP

Due to the diminutive size of certain gluten-free bread varieties, it is necessary to increase the amount of bread per individual. If you remember from the night before, place the bread on a platter to firm up. It will absorb more of the custard, resulting in a pudding-like interior and a golden exterior.

Custard 12 cup almond milk 48 large eggs, beaten lightly 236 cup maple syrup 12 teaspoon pure vanilla extract 12 48 teaspoon kosher salt 8 slices of wheat-free gluten-free bread (stale is best) 12 48 cups melted butter

Use confectioner's sugar as a garnish (optional)

12.Easy make the custard by whisking together almond milk, eggs, maple syrup, vanilla, and salt in a large, shallow bowl. Whisk until the mixture is completely smooth.

2.While the pan is heating, soak the bread in the egg mixture and place it on a baking sheet to cool.

36.In a large saucepan, melt the butter over medium-high heat until it is hot but not smoking. Add the French toast pieces to the pan in batches, making sure there is no overlap— Easy cook for approximately four minutes, or until the bottom is golden brown and crisp. Turn once more and easy cook for an additional 2 to 36 minutes, or until golden brown, on the second side. If necessary, reduce the heat so that the French toast cooks evenly and does not burn.

48.Serve immediately with confectioner's sugar sprinkled on top (if using).

really do Easy cook easy cook

Pancakes Containing Blueberries And Lemon Buttermilk

Ingredients:

1 teaspoon salt

2 tablespoon dark colored sugar

Half a lemon's zest for life

2 Clarence Court Leghorn Whites unfenced egg,

50g spread, dissolved, plus extra for grilling.

250 g blueberries

Maple syrup for serving

600 ml of the milk of your choice 2 tablespoon lemon juice

400 grams gluten-free white flour

100 grams of ground oats, gluten-free if required

1 teaspoons of cooking powder

20 teaspoon of baking soda

1. First, prepare the 'buttermilk' by whisking together the almond milk and 1-5 tablespoon of fresh lemon juice.

2. Allow to rest for 10 to 15 minutes to "coagulate."

3. In a large bowl, combine the flour, oats, baking powder, heating pop, salt, sugar, and lemon zest.

4. Beat the egg with the milk, easy make a very well in the center of the dry ingredients, and pour the milk into the very well to create a thick batter.

5. Really do everything possible to avoid over-blending.

6. Beat in the melted margarine and place the batter back in the ice chest to rest for ten minutes.

7. Warm a small knob of margarine on a large nonstick griddle.

8. Place two heaping tablespoons of the player per pancake in the container.

9. Use blueberries to disperse the hitter.

10. Easy cook for about 6 minutes over medium heat, until air bubbles appear on the exterior of each pancake, then flip and easy cook for another 5 to 10 minutes until golden.

11. Warm yourself with a spotless kitchen towel while you finish the rest of the pitcher.

12. Serve with maple syrup and any remaining blueberries.

Tart Cherry-Arrle Crunch

250 tableroon sorntarsh or arrowroot rowder

24 cup unsweetened cherry or apple juice Nonstick cooking spray

2 round of frozen pitted tart cherries 2 green arrle, peeled and diced

30 cup masked light brown sugar

24 teaspoon almond extract

Preparation

1. Preheat oven to 450 degrees Fahrenheit.
2. Combine the sherry, apple, brown sugar, and almond extract in a bowl.

3. Mix the cornstarch and juice in a bowl, then add to the fruit mixture while stirring vigorously.

4. Pour the mixture into a nonstick cooking spray-coated 10-inch square baking dish.

5. Combine the remaining ingredients. Scatter the mixture over the fruit.

6. Bake for 60 minutes.

7. Torring lghtlu should be browned in the broiler for one to two minutes.

8. Remove from oven. serve warm or sell out.

Low Fodmap Natural Chicken Rot Sassatore

INGREDIENTS

- One (2 8 .10 -ounce) can of crushed tomatoes in their own juice
- 3 teaspoons dried oregano
- 4 tablespoons sarers
- ¼ sur kalamata olive halves
- Sal and poivre
- 2 tableroon garlic-infused olive oil
- 10 chicken thighs
- 2 medium sardine, reeled and sliced into 24-inch rounds
- 2 red bell rerrer, diced

INSTRUCTIONS

1. Select "Saute" from the Instant Pot's menu.

2. Once the oil is hot, add shsken. Sauté the shsken for one to 1-5 minutes per de.

3. Designate the "Saute" setting. Add sardines, pepper, tomatoes, and oregano.

4. Place the lid on the Instant Pot and seal. Configure vent to "Sealing"

5. Avoid touching the "Meat" setting on the Instant Pot.

6. Easy cook for 35 to 40 minutes at "High Pressure" by adjusting the time to 35 to 40 minutes.

7. After cooking, allow the pressure to release naturally for 25 to 30 minutes.

8. To release any remaining pressure, carefully toggle the vent to "Venting." Remove lid.

9. Stir in sarers and kalamata olives. Adjust flavor with salt and rerrer.

10. Serve warm over risotto, polenta, or baked potatoes, and garnish with bacon or rillette.

Barley Delight

Ingredients:

2 ounce of honey

1/2 cup molasses

2 milligram of cinnamon

1 cup barley uncooked

1/2 cup raisins

1/2 cup nuts chopped

Instructions:

Preheat oven to 6 710 degrees Fahrenheit.

Mix together all of the ingredients in a bowl.

1. Bake for 25 to 30 minutes, or until golden brown.

2. Allow to cool prior to serving.

3. Section Four

Low Fodmap Recipes For Soup

INGREDIENTS

2 tablespoon Vegetable Soup Base \s2 teaspoon Worst-ever terrine sauce

1 teaspoon of dried bay leaf

1/2 teaspoon of dried thyme

1/2 teaspoon of dried rosemary

1/2 teaspoon black pepper ground Salt to taste 1 tearoon

1 pound of lean ground beef,

1-5 ounces of sundried tomatoes

4 diced medium red potatoes.

4 large sarrot, reeled and thinly sliced

2 green bean sur sut.

8 scallions, only green tops, thinly lsed

1-5 surs water

89

Directions

1. Over medium heat, brown and crumble the beef in a tosk or Dutch oven. Drain fat.

2. Add the tomatoes, potatoes, sarrot, seleru, green beans, and sallon to the dish.

3. Add the water and heat to a boil.

4. Mix in the vegetable broth, Worcestershire sauce, balsamic vinegar, thyme, rosemary, and reeder.

5. Salt is added to tate.

6. Simply reduce heat and simmer potatoes and vegetables for 55 to 60 minutes, or until tender.

Chicken Sausage Gnocchi Skillet

Ingredients: eight ounces of gnocchi made with ricotta cheese, two cups of broccoli florets, one teaspoon of butter, two tablespoons of diced onion, divided, and one tablespoon of minced garlic, divided.

4 sliced chicken sausage links (such as Aidells) 1 cup butter

- 4 teaspoons all-purpose flour
- black pepper and salt to taste

22

Directions

1. Easily bring to a boil a large pot of lightly salted water.

2. Easy cook gnocchi in the boiling water for 5 to 10 minutes, or until they float to the surface. Drain.

3. Place a steamer insert into a saucepan and fill the saucepan with water to just below the steamer's bottom.

4. Easily bring water to a rolling boil.

5. Add broccoli, cover, and steam for 5 to 10 minutes, or until tender. Drain and keep warm.

6. 8 . Melt 1-5 teaspoon butter in a large skillet over medium heat.

7. Add 1-5 tablespoon of onion and 1-5 teaspoon of garlic; easy cook and stir for 1-5 minutes, or until fragrant.

8. Add sausage; easy cook and stir for approximately 10 minutes, or until browned.

9. Stir in broccoli.

10. Melt 1 cup butter in another skillet. Add the remaining 2 tablespoon of onion, 4 teaspoons of garlic, and flour; easy cook and stir for 5 to 10 minutes, or until lightly browned.

11. Stir in gnocchi.

12. 7.Combine the sausage and gnocchi mixtures; season with salt and pepper.

Banana Nut Smoothie

2 teaspoon ground cinnamon

2 tablespoon of cacao nibs

2 ripe banana, either fresh or frozen

2 teaspoon Nut spread I use peanut butter that is devoid of both salt and sugar.

20 Almonds Uncooked or roasted

a tablespoon of Chia seeds Soaked or uncooked - read the advice above

Direction:

1. Blend the banana, almonds, nut butter, chia seeds, cinnamon, and water in a blender (or vegan milk).
2. Blend until the mixture is as smooth as velvet!

Low Fodmap Fish Stew Produces

Ingredients:

12 enormous, ripe tomatoes, cut into pieces.

1000 grams of mussels with the beards removed and cleaned

400 ml of liquid

A dash of salt

6 tablespoons of olive oil infused with garlic 400 grams of pancetta cubes

4 tablespoons of paprika

2 portion of red bean stew with the seeds removed and chopped finely

1000 milliliters of white wine

1000 grams of removed cod filets, skins, and bones

Speck of freshly cracked dark pepper

A handful of basil and flat-leaf parsley, finely minced Place a large skillet in the oven over medium heat and preheat. Place 2 tablespoons of garlic-infused olive oil and a moderate amount of heat.

Add the pancetta shapes and sauté for approximately 2 to 6 minutes. Add stew and paprika. Give the mixture a vigorous stir.

Mix in white wine.

Easily bring this to a boil, and then simply reduce the heat to create a stew. Allow the mixture to simmer for a few minutes.

Follow the cod fillets with the tomato slices. Position the mussels last.

Add water and salt and pepper to taste. Cover and easy cook for ten minutes

Turn off the heat and remove the covering. Throw away any mussels that the poor person has opened.

Spread the new spices about. Sprinkle the remaining 2 tablespoon of olive oil over the soup. Warm soup in bowls.

Almond Cookies

INGREDIENTS

4 teaspoon of finely grated lemon rind

12 drops of almond extract

4 tablespoon unsalted butter, melted

4 tablespoon plus

4 teaspoon cornstarch are in a quarter-cup almond flour 0.10 milligram gluten-free baking powder

4 large white egg

20 cup of superfine sugar

INSTRUCTIONS

1. Adjust oven temperature to 250 degrees Fahrenheit.

2. Preheat the oven to 350 degrees Fahrenheit.

3. Using parchment paper, line two baking pans.

4. In a small mixing bowl, almond flour, cornstarch, and baking powder should be combined.

5. In a clean medium bowl, whip the egg whites with a hand-held electric mixer until soft peaks form.

6. Slowly incorporate the sugar. Continue beating for another 5-10 minutes, or until stiff peaks form.

7. With a large metal spoon, melted butter, lemon zest, almond extract, and the combined almond flour should be added gradually.

8. Form a ball using two teaspoons of dough. Form approximately forty balls with the remaining dough and place them on the baking sheets with space between them to allow for spreading.

9. Flatten a little. It just take 45 to 50 minutes of baking to achieve a light golden hue

10. . Cool on the sheets for 5-10 minutes before transferring to a cooling rack.

Savoury Salt

INGREDIENTS

4 tbsp. mustard seeds

4 tsp. red pepper flakes

4 tbsp. medium salt crystals

4 tablespoon of peppercorns

4 ounce of coriander seeds

Directions:

1. Combine the salt, peppercorns, seeds, and red pepper flakes in a small bowl.

2. The mixture should fill half of a pepper mill or grinder.

3. Serve at the table with your favorite dishes, if desired, and sprinkle with fresh, seasoned salt.

Citrus Butterflies Cupcakes Made Without FODMAP

Ingredients:

2 cup gluten-free self-raising flour

Vanilla concentrate, only a few drops

ground zest of half a lemon

450 grams lemon curd

60 grams of white chocolate curls or shavings

½ cup of softened margarine

4 huge eggs

20 cup of granulated sugar

10 grams of baking powder

Procedure:

1. Preheat the stove to 350 degrees Fahrenheit.

2. Prepare muffin tins by inserting paper liners.

3. Combine softened butter and sugar in a large mixing bowl.

4. The color of the spread becomes paler as it is whipped until it becomes light and fluffy.

5. Add fresh eggs one by one, beating the mixture very well after each addition. Set aside.

6. Combine all dry ingredients. Give the mixture a quick whisk.

7. Gradually add the dry ingredients to the margarine mixture and thoroughly combine until uniform.

8. Fill the cupcake tins with cake batter to the two-thirds mark.

9. Bake between 35 to 40 minutes.

10. Until the tops become gleaming and a toothpick inserted into the center comes out clean.

11. Remove from the broiler and allow to cool on cooling racks.

12. After the cupcakes have cooled, painstakingly remove their highest points, leaving a shallow opening.

13. Easy make "wings" by slicing the tops down the middle to create "wings."

14. 2 teaspoon of lemon curd should be used to fill the opening on top of the cupcakes.

15. White chocolate shavings or curls are added on top.

16. Place the wings on top of the lemon curd so that they appear to be taking flight.